The No-Shame Parent

Promoting Open Communication and Trust

Table of Contents

Chapter 1. Introduction

Dive into a refreshingly honest exploration of modern parenting with our Special Report: "The No-Shame Parent: Promoting Open Communication and Trust". This guide is your ticket to evolving your parenting skills in this dynamic world, providing you with powerful insights and actionable strategies to create a shame-free environment at home. Foster open communication lines with your child, and build a unshakeable bond based on mutual respect and trust. This is not just a report; it's an opportunity to transform your parenthood journey into a liberating, joyful, and inclusive experience. If this sounds like the kind of journey you'd like to embark upon, then this Special Report is just a click away. Get yours today, and rekindle the beautiful, loving relationship you deserve with your child!

Chapter 2. Understanding the No-Shame Parenting Approach

The no-shame parenting approach is much more than a catchphrase; it's a philosophy and a methodology centered around respect, understanding, mutual admiration, and above all, effective communication sans any form of shaming and critical judgments. The aim is to establish a profound connection with your child while steering their development in a positive direction.

2.1. The Essence of No-Shame Parenting

At its core, no-shame parenting embraces the concept of responsivity - the ability to react appropriately and positively to a child's emotional needs. The focus shifts from scoring discipline points to understanding the inherent emotions and assisting in developing the essential skills needed to regulate these emotions. Instead of shaming and embarrassing the child for their wrongdoings, parents adopting this approach aim to guide their child through the situation, helping them understand the implications of their actions without belittling their feelings or thoughts.

Shaming children often leads to a negative self-image and a drop in self-esteem, which inhibits their overall development. No-shame parenting encourages parents to educate their children on right and wrong, fostering a healthy perception of self, others, and the world around them.

2.2. The Importance of Positive Communication

Communication sits at the heart of no-shame parenting. However, the accent here is on 'positive' communication. It's crucial to show your child that you're not just the authority figure in their life but a friend and confidant with whom they can share their fears, aspirations, and experiences without any fear of judgment.

Avoiding negative language, not jumping to conclusions, and listening actively are a few strategies you can employ. Remember, maintaining open channels of communication doesn't mean agreeing with every decision your child makes. Instead, it's about understanding their viewpoint, appreciating their feelings, and guiding them towards mindful decision-making.

2.3. Teaching Responsibility Without Resorting to Shame

An important aspect of no-shame parenting is instilling a sense of responsibility in children. Traditional parenting often conflates shaming with teaching responsibility, using guilt to coerce children into shouldering responsibilities. However, in the no-shame parenting approach, responsibility equates more with understanding the consequences of one's actions and making amends if required.

Instead of reprimanding your child for their mistakes, guide them on understanding the mistake, realizing its impact, and identifying ways to set things right. This method not only imparts responsibility but also instills an innate ability to self-correct and comprehend the consequences of their actions.

2.4. Encouraging Emotional Expression

Traditional parenting often stifles emotional expression, viewing it as a sign of weakness. However, no-shame parenting champions emotional expression, recognizing that it fosters emotional intelligence

Conversations about feelings should be a commonplace occurrence in your household, whether they revolve around joy, sadness, anger, or fear. The idea is to not suppress these emotions but to understand and express them appropriately. Teach your child that no emotion is 'good' or 'bad'; instead, let them know it's the response to these emotions that they can control and manage.

2.5. Cultivating a Culture of Empathy

Empathy forms the crux of no-shame parenting as it builds a two-way street of understanding and respect. Empathize with your child's struggles and situations, creating a climate of emotional safety. Show your child that it's okay to have a bad day, it's okay to make a mistake, and it's okay to be imperfect.

In turn, teach your child about empathy. Show them how to relate to others' feelings and let them experience firsthand the positive impacts of empathetic actions. This will not only strengthen your bond but also equip your child with valuable skills that will help in their personal and social interactions.

2.6. Building Strong Relationships with Trust

Trust serves as the landing gear of the flight to no-shame parenting, creating an environment where the child feels safe and secure. Upholding your promises, setting realistic expectations, and leading by example are ways of establishing trust.

The aim is to make your child feel that they can count on you for support, guidance, and love. Over time, your child will mirror these trust-building behaviors, carving a pathway to genuine, enduring relationships.

No-shame parenting is a compassionate journey focused on encouraging growth, open communication, emotional expression while shunning shaming, judgement, and guilt. As you move towards becoming a no-shame parent, you'll discover not just a resilient bond with your child, but also a refreshing perspective on parenthood itself. This report is your map- walk the journey and cherish the transformation at every step.

Chapter 3. Building Blocks of Trust in Parent-Child Relationships

Trust is an intangible asset but carries incredible weight in influencing the nature of every human relationship, most importantly the relationship between a parent and a child. A strong, healthy bond paved with trust provides a solid foundation for your child to grow, learn, and brave the challenges life presents.

3.1. The Essence of Trust

Trust is a robust and essential layer that imbues a relationship with honesty, familiarity, security, and love. In the context of a parent-child relationship, trust becomes even more crucial, as children look towards their parents as their first and most influential role models. It is the lens through which children perceive the world. Building trust is akin to shaping this lens, which can imbue them with confidence and compassion, or conversely, with fear and skepticism.

Building trust with your children involves showing them consistently that they can depend on you for their needs and wants. It requires you to demonstrate to them that you are reliable and predictable. When you say you'll do something - you follow through. This shows your child that they can rely on you, fostering trust.

Trust is not a static state, but rather a dynamic, ever-changing entity influenced by your actions, reactions, and inactions as a parent. It requires continuous nurturing and, at times, mending. Trust, once broken, is not easily regained, highlighting the importance and responsibility involved in maintaining it.

3.2. Establishing Trust in Early Years

The journey to establishing trust starts from the early years of your child's life. Infants and toddlers, despite their limited understanding, can sense your emotional state and rely on your consistency to feel secure.

During this stage, regularity and dependability in routines, like feeding, sleeping, and play time, help to foster trust. By ensuring that your child's basic needs are taken care of on a predictable schedule, you instill in them a sense of safety and reliability, thus strengthening their trust in you.

This early bond of trust forms the foundation for your child's social, emotional, and cognitive development. It influences their ability to form secure relationships in the future, their self-esteem, and their readiness to learn and explore the world.

3.3. Nurturing Trust through Open Communication

As your child grows older, the methods to foster trust evolve. While dependability continues to be crucial, open communication becomes increasingly significant.

Engaging in regular conversation with your child, taking an interest in their thoughts, feelings, and experiences, and offering understanding and support, all contribute to a trusting environment. As a parent, endeavor to be proactive in your communication. It's essential to let your child know that their voice is welcomed and that their feelings are valid.

Strive to maintain a verbal and non-verbal communication balance with your child. The tone of your voice, your body language, and your facial expressions, should all reflect your openness and willingness to engage.

Moreover, honesty is paramount. There may be times when you feel the urge to shield your child from certain truths due to their age or the issue's sensitivity. However, always remember that delicately explained honesty outweighs deception. Honesty strengthens trust and makes your child feel respected and included.

3.4. Encouraging Emotional Expressiveness

Trust, to a great extent, is rooted in emotional transparency and validation. Encouraging your child to freely express their feelings and emotions and providing validation promotes trust. Make it a habit to discuss emotions at home, both good and challenging ones.

When your child opens up about their feelings, even if their reactions seem overblown or unreasonable to you, it's crucial that you never minimize or dismiss them. Hear them out, and validate their feelings. Teach them that it's okay to feel what they feel and that they can share their feelings with you without fear of judgment or ridicule.

3.5. Handling Mistakes with Care

Children, as they grow, are bound to make mistakes and poor choices. It is an essential part of their growth and learning, but mishandling such situations can strain trust.

When your child makes a mistake, it provides an opportunity to bolster trust by showcasing your love, understanding, and guidance. Instead of anger or punishment, opt for calmness and education. Such an approach reassures them that they are loved, irrespective of their actions or decisions.

3.6. Consistent Behavior and Actions

Your actions and behavior have a significant impact on your child's trust in you. Ensure that you always follow through on what you say, as children are keen observers. If you promise a reward or a consequence, follow through. This consistency helps build trust as it shows your child that you mean what you say.

3.7. Respecting Boundaries

Recognizing and respecting your child's boundaries is an often overlooked aspect of building trust. Everyone has personal boundaries, and children are no exception. Respecting their boundaries conveys to them that their comfort, privacy and opinions are valuable to you, thereby fostering trust.

Building trust is not a destination but a journey. It is a continuous process of providing love and security, encouraging open communication, validating emotions, handling mistakes appropriately, being consistent, and respecting boundaries. Despite the efforts required, the profoundly positive impact it has on your child, their personality and your relationship with them, makes this journey extremely rewarding.

Chapter 4. The Power of Open Communication: A Step-by-Step Guide

Communicating with your children can sometimes seem like navigating a maze—full of winding paths, dead ends, and sudden turns. Understanding the importance of open communication is one of the vital steps to successful modern parenting.

4.1. The Pivot Towards Open Communication

Our society churns at a hectic speed. The exponential growth in technology, coupled with the constant flux in societal norms, makes parenting a complex task. In this dynamic environment, open two-way communication is indispensable. It goes beyond talking and listening; it's about understanding, empathy, and connection.

Open communication isn't a novelty; it's a necessity, a pivot that we must turn towards. Why? Because it fuels the parent-child relationship, fostering an environment of trust, understanding, and respect. It helps you empathize with your child's worldview, understand the skirmish of feelings they experience, and provide them with a safe space to express their fears or ideas without judgment.

Conversely, open communication enhances your child's confidence, enhances their emotional intelligence, and equips them with the ability to navigate the world and foster healthy relationships.

4.2. Understanding the Components of Open Communication

Open communication comprises three key components:

1. Active Listening: An attentive and receptive form of listening where you fully concentrate, understand, respond, and remember what is being said.

2. Empathy: It's about understanding and sharing the feelings of your child, getting out of your shoes, and walking around in theirs.

3. Constructive Response: This is effectively responding to the communication, offering support, understanding, and guidance without criticism or bias.

These components form the very foundation that lets the structure of open communication stand strong and firm.

4.3. The Roadmap to Open Communication

Here's a step-by-step guide to incorporate open communication in your parenthood journey:

1. Start Early: Early childhood is an opportune time to lay the groundwork for open communication. Use simple language, talk about their day, read aloud, and encourage them to express their thoughts and feelings.

2. Active Listening: Listen not just to respond, but to understand. This means not interrupting, offering your undivided attention, and thinking before you respond. Also, interpret their non-verbal cues.

3. Talk Their Interests: Engage in discussions about their interests. It might be dinosaurs, ballet, or a favorite TV show. This shows your interest in their world and prompts them to share more.

4. Regular Conversation Times: Dinner tables, bedtime stories, or car rides can be inculcated as 'conversation zones' where everyone shares their day or discusses any topic.

5. Ask Open-Ended Questions: Asking questions that do not elicit a 'yes' or 'no' response encourages your child to think and express their thoughts.

6. Respect Their Opinions: Respect their thoughts and ideas, no matter how different they are from yours. This shows that you value their opinions.

7. Be Humble: By admitting your mistakes, you create an environment where it's okay to be wrong and learn from it.

8. Show Empathy: Connect with their emotions, validate them, even if they seem trivial.

9. Keep a Check on Your Reactions: Avoid any kind of judgment, sarcasm, or anger in your responses. It hinders open communication.

10. Encourage Feedback: Encourage them to express how they feel about your guidance or parenting style.

4.4. Persistence is Key

Remember that open communication is not an overnight shift—it's a steady glide. At times, the road may seem unending or strenuous, but persistence is critical.

And never forget, communication is a two-way street—sometimes you talk, many times you listen. But when this conversation flows without judgment set against the backdrop of love, trust, and respect, it forms the essence of open communication—the beautiful dance of parenthood.

Chapter 5. Creating a Shame-Free Home: Practical Tips and Techniques

Raising children in a shame-free environment is not just a desire of every parent, it also forms the foundation of a healthy child-adult relationship. In this endeavor, it's imperative to follow an open, honest, and communicative approach while dealing with children.

5.1. Understanding Shame

The journey towards creating a shame-free home begins with understanding what shame entails. Shame is a deeply ingrained emotion that can lead to a person feeling 'flawed,' 'wrong,' or 'unworthy.' When children perceive these feelings, their self-esteem and self-worth are heavily impacted, often leading to long-term psychological effects. It's crucial to remember that all children, regardless of age, are prone to feeling shame–but the good news is parents can do a lot to curtail or notably lessen this.

5.2. Cultivate Emotional Intelligence

Encouraging emotional intelligence is a significant first step to ensure a shame-free environment. Enable your child to recognize, understand, and articulate their feelings. Be patient and allow them space for processing their emotions during conversations. You may begin with leading questions like, 'You seem upset. Do you want to talk about it?' This can make the child more comfortable expressing their feelings, reducing the chance of inducing shame.

5.3. Promote Open and Honest Communication

Open communication forms the backbone of a trusting parent-child relationship. Make it a point to engage in daily conversations with your child–about their day, their likes or dislikes, their concerns or worries, their small achievements, or their dreams. Such conversations should ideally be conducted within neutral environments–perhaps a walk in the park, during a drive, or over a meal. This not only encourages your child to voice out feelings but also reassures them that what they share will not be judged or punished.

5.4. Normalize Failure and Encourage Resilience

Even on the most challenging days, stay away from blaming or shaming your child for their failures. Instead, normalize these setbacks and treat them as stepping stones to success. Teach your child to embrace their mistakes as learning opportunities. Encouraging phrases like, 'I'm proud of you for trying..' or 'Let's figure out another way to do this...' can help in building their resilience.

5.5. Fostering Cooperative Behavior

In a shame-free home, rules and boundaries must be presented as tools for harmonious living rather than oppressive orders. This can be achieved by discussing and involving the child in the rule-setting process, thereby making them understand their responsibility towards maintaining peace and harmony at home.

5.6. Swapping Punishment with Natural Consequences

A shame-free home does not mean a discipline-free home. However, traditional punitive measures should be replaced with natural consequences. For example, if a child refuses to do their homework, the natural consequence may be poor grades. You may explain this correlation to your child, without blaming or shaming them for their action.

5.7. Practice Non-Violent Communication

Non-violent communication ensures respect, empathy, and compassion–crucial elements in building a shame-free home. Parents must learn to frame requests instead of orders, express their feelings without accusation, and listen actively to their child's needs and concerns.

5.8. Surround Your Child with Positive Affirmations

Language matters! Choose your words carefully when interacting with your child, avoiding harmful labels or name-calling. Instead, use positive affirmations and appreciative phrases that boost their confidence and self-esteem.

5.9. Be a Role Model

Remember, children learn more from what you do than what you say. Displaying empathy, honesty, resilience, and forgiveness in your actions can inspire your child to embody these characteristics.

5.10. Seek Professional Guidance If Necessary

Lastly, don't hesitate to seek professional help if you notice persistent signs of shame or low self-esteem in your child. A trained professional can assist your family in understanding and managing these feelings.

In conclusion, creating a shame-free home is an ongoing process that requires conscious effort, patience, and adaptability. It's not an overnight task but a commitment to fostering and nurturing an atmosphere of mutual respect, understanding, and love.

Chapter 6. Parenting in the Digital Age: Challenges and Opportunities

Twenty-first century parenting is a world apart from what it was a few decades ago. The advent of digital technology and its pervasive influence on all aspects of life has added a new dimension to parenting, bringing with it unique challenges as well as unexplored opportunities.

6.1. Digital Expansion: The World at Your Fingertips

The rise of the Internet, smartphones, and social media have revolutionized our daily lives. Children nowadays are digital natives, born and raised surrounded by technology. With just a click or a screen tap, a broad plethora of information, entertainment, and social interaction is accessible at their fingertips. The digital world is their playground, an all-encompassing expanse where they explore, learn, and grow. While this digital playground exposes children to an infinite scope of knowledge, it also brings about the unfortunate side-effects of screen addiction, cyberbullying, inappropriate content, and digital privacy issues.

6.2. Striking the Right Balance: Screen Time Management

One of the significant challenges parents face is managing their children's screen time. Studies indicate that excessive screen use can affect a child's mental and physical health. Establishing healthy screen time habits requires parents to create guidelines, enforce breaks, and engage in shared media use. Parental control apps can be beneficial tools, helping parents monitor and manage children's digital consumption. However, remember, the goal is to instill self-regulation and not create an atmosphere of surveillance.

6.3. Cyberbullying and Online Safety

The digital age has spawned a new form of bullying – 'Cyberbullying'. With almost every child active on social media platforms, they are susceptible to harassment, intimidation, or humiliation. Talking openly about the potential dangers, encouraging children to discuss their online experiences, and teaching them appropriate online behavior can help create a secure digital environment. Employing simple strategies like adjusting privacy settings, regularly checking friend lists, and reporting abusive behavior can considerably enhance online safety.

6.4. Evading the Digital Pitfalls

While internet safety is of paramount concern to parents, avoiding internet-related challenges doesn't merely involve putting up defenses. An essential aspect of navigating the digital world is understanding its language, knowing the apps, games, and social platforms your children partake in. Staying informed allows parents to anticipate issues before they arise and provide the right guidance when children encounter challenging digital situations.

6.5. Harnessing the Power of Technology for Education

Technology isn't just fun and games. The digital age brings an ocean of educational opportunities that modern parents can leverage. E-books, online tutorials, educational apps, and virtual reality learning are redefining the traditional concept of learning. The key lies in using these tools effectively to enhance a child's understanding and curiosity. Parents should stay involved, observe their child's progress, and ensure the tech tools align with their learning objectives.

6.6. Building a Digital Code of Conduct

Developing a digital code of conduct is imperative in this age. This code can be a set of norms that reflects shared values and expectations around digital technology use. A successful code of conduct should include privacy, etiquette, time management, and the obligation to discuss any inappropriate content or uncomfortable online interactions.

6.7. Technology Teaches Responsibility

While technology poses challenges, it also creates an avenue for teaching responsibility. Assigning children a particular device or a digital task can help instill a sense of ownership and responsibility. They can learn to manage gadget maintenance, use tech tools responsibly, and respect the privacy of others online.

6.8. Fostering Real Connections in a Digital World

In this digital age, fostering real connections and face-to-face interactions is essential for a child's socio-emotional development. Encourage activities that involve interpersonal engagement—family outings, get-togethers with friends, and participation in clubs or sports. Life beyond screens should be equally, if not more, vibrant and fulfilling as the virtual world.

Parenting in the digital age may appear daunting with morphing digital landscapes and emerging cyber threats. However, with informed strategies and open communication, parents can convert these challenges into opportunities. It's about facilitating your child's digital journey, keeping them safe while allowing them to harness the full potential of digital technology in a responsible and meaningful way.

Chapter 7. Listening Skills for No-Shame Parenting

Successful parenting requires active and perceptive listening. When you listen to your children properly—even when they're expressing anger or anxiety—you validate their emotions without casting judgment, nurturing a safe and shame-free environment for communication.

7.1. The Art of Active Listening

Active listening is an integral part of effective communication, especially with children. This process involves not just hearing their words, but understanding their thoughts and feelings.

For active listening, you should strive to stay engaged, maintain eye contact, provide confirming nods, and use affirmations like "I understand" or "That must be tough." These small actions communicate to the child that you're genuinely interested in what they're saying. Active listening fosters a sense of worthiness in them and reassures them that their feelings matter.

7.2. Cultivate Empathy in Communication

To truly understand and connect with your child, you should cultivate empathy in your communication. Empathy involves imagining yourself in your child's situation, genuinely feeling their emotions, and then responding with care. It could mean something as simple as acknowledging their feelings, "It must be really hard to lose a game you practiced so hard for."

7.3. Encourage Open Expressions

Regularly seek opportunities to talk with your child. Create an environment where they can come to you with any issue, without fear of judgment or shame. This approach strengthens your bond and helps you proactively address any emotional or behavioral concerns.

7.4. Nurturing Emotional Literacy

Emotional literacy—understanding and expressing feelings—enables us to communicate effectively. As parents, promote emotional literacy by teaching your child to name their feelings and recognise them in others. It anticipates the risk of miscommunication and misunderstanding.

7.5. From Reactivity to Responsivity

A no-shame parenting approach involves shifting from a reactive stance—one that can be dominated by knee-jerk reactions and punishments—to a responsive one. In a responsive stance, you strive to understand underlying feelings, needs, or triggers behind your child's behavior and filter your responses through this understanding.

7.6. Validation, Not minimization

When a child comes to you with a concern or problem, try to avoid dismissing or minimizing their feelings. Instead, validate their feelings as genuine by expressing that it's alright to feel the way they do.

7.7. Building Trust Through Listening

Trust is the cornerstone of any relationship, including the one with your child. One of the best ways to build trust in your relationship is to truly listen when they speak. You need to make an effort to drop everything and give them your undivided attention when they come to you.

With these practices in mind, embracing active listening can significantly enrich your parenting journey, paving the way for a shame-free nurturing environment. After all, our greatest goal as parents is to cultivate a healthy and positive relationship with our children which can stand the test of time and life's many challenges.

Chapter 8. Dealing with Peer Pressure and Bullying: A Parent's Guide

Peer pressure and bullying have been issues of concern for generations. Despite the awareness and measures in place to combat these challenges, they continue to persist in new shapes and forms, becoming ever-more complex in the light of digital advancements. As parents, it becomes our duty not only to protect our children from such harmful external influences but also to equip them with the required social-emotional skills to manoeuvre through such situations by themselves.

8.1. Understanding Peer Pressure

Understanding is the first step towards resolution. Peer pressure, in essence, is the influence that a peer group, observers or an individual exerts, which encourages others to change their attitudes, values, or behaviours to conform to those of the influencing group or individual. It can manifest both positively and negatively.

Positive peer pressure encourages constructive habits like studying, participating in physical activities, volunteering, and refraining from detrimental behaviours. Negative peer pressure, on the other hand, can lead to harmful activities such as substance abuse, inappropriate conduct and unhealthy risk-taking.

8.2. The Influence of Negative Peer Pressure

Negative peer pressure often intensifies during the adolescent years of a child when their desire for independence and acceptance from their social circle peaks. They might yield to the pressure to fit in, trying to avoid feelings of rejection, humiliation or a sense of being left out.

The influence can often manifest in actions such as cheating, lying, skipping school, experimenting with drugs or alcohol, or becoming sexually active at an early age. These unfair expectations and influences can cause significant levels of stress, confusion, and fear.

Therefore, as a first step, it is pivotal to nurture an open communication channel with your child about these matters.

8.3. Addressing Negative Peer Pressure

1. **Open Dialogue** : Begin by maintaining an open channel for conversation with your child. This will not only keep you aware of their activities and thoughts but also make them feel comfortable coming to you when they face any issues.

2. **Encourage good friendships** : Promote healthy friendships and encourage spending time with peers who possess positive values, offering a good influence.

3. **Build Self-esteem** : Encourage and appreciate your child to build their self-confidence. Encourage them to pursue interests and activities that make them feel good about themselves, fostering the belief that they don't need to conform to other's expectations.

8.4. Understanding Bullying

Bullying is harmful, aggressive behaviour instigated by one or more individuals towards another individual on repeated occasions. This could be physical (hitting, pushing), verbal (teasing, calling names), and increasingly, online, also known as cyber-bullying.

An understanding and readiness to tackle bullying are essential for the safety, confidence, and overall well-being of your child.

8.5. The Impact of Bullying

Studies have shown that children who are bullied experience real suffering that can interfere with their social and emotional development, as well as their school performance. They can develop a range of symptoms from depression, anxiety, low self-esteem, health problems, and even suicidal thoughts in extreme cases.

Therefore, it is crucial for every parent to understand the gravity of this issue and create a supportive environment at home to counter these experiences.

8.6. Addressing Bullying

1. **Recognize the signs**: The first step to address bullying involves recognizing the signs. Unexplainable injuries, loss of personal items, decreased appetite, frequent nightmares are telltale signs that a child might be the victim of bullying.

2. **Open communication**: Ensure to have regular conversations with your child about their school life, friendships, and any unusual incidents. Establish trust in the communication such that they feel comfortable speaking up when needed.

3. **Empower your child**: Involve your child in decisions concerning bully-prevention strategies. Simple responses or walking away can stop further bullying, as it halts the Bully's intended reaction.

4. **Get School Authorities involved**: If your child is being bullied in school, it is important to get the school administration involved to address this serious issue collectively.

5. **Promote empathy**: Encourage kindness, empathy and involve them in activities that teach social and emotional learning,

building their emotional intelligence.

In conclusion, the prevalence and impact of peer pressure and bullying on young minds cannot be taken lightly and needs to be addressed proactively. As parents, our role expands beyond just ensuring their basic comfort. It also involves creating an environment that nurtures confident, empathetic and resilient individuals equipped to confront the challenges of today's world.

Chapter 9. Promoting Resilience and Emotional Intelligence in Children

Resilience and emotional intelligence are critical skills in the world today. Reinforcing these skills in children can help them to flourish in challenging environments and to bounce back from disappointments, setbacks, and failures.

9.1. Understanding Resilience

Resilience is not just about bouncing back; it is about bending without breaking and staying adaptive under pressure. It's about learning to cope with problems, adapting to changes and recovering from adversity. Children who develop resilience at a young age are better equipped to tackle problems and bounce back from failures and disappointments.

Resilience can be fostered in children, regardless of their personality or age. It involves teaching them problem-solving skills, nurturing a positive self-view, emotional regulation, and helping them to create and maintain supportive relationships.

9.2. Strategies to Foster Resilience

Practice has proven that resilience can be nurtured and developed. Here are few strategies you can employ to foster resilience in your child:

Encourage Problem-Solving Skills: It's natural to want to solve your child's problems, but children need to experience challenges to develop problem-solving capabilities. Allow your child to suffer manageable consequences of their actions. This will provide your child with the experience necessary to learn from their mistakes and develop problem-solving skills.

Promote a Positive Self-View: It's crucial to help your child develop a positive understanding of their abilities. Encourage your child to recognize their strengths and weaknesses and to value their own unique skills and qualities. This helps build their self-esteem and resilience.

Nurture Supportive Relationships: Develop strong, warm relationships, both within the family and outside of it. Robust social connections can foster a sense of belonging and security, enhancing resilience.

9.3. Understanding Emotional Intelligence

Emotional intelligence, often abbreviated as EI or EQ, is a person's ability to understand and manage their own emotions and the emotions of others. It involves skills like emotional awareness, the ability to apply emotions to problem-solving, emotional regulation, and empathy.

High levels of EI are associated with better communication skills, improved relationships, self-confidence, and better coping capabilities for stress and challenges.

9.4. Strategies to Develop Emotional Intelligence

Developing emotional intelligence in children is possible with consistent practice. Here are a few strategies to foster EI:

Teach Emotional Awareness: Teach your child to identify their emotions and the emotions of others. Use everyday experiences to discuss emotions.

Encourage Expression of Emotions: Encourage your child to express their feelings verbally. Support them in using appropriate words to describe how they feel. This builds a rich emotional vocabulary and helps them communicate effectively.

Teach Emotional Regulation: Teach your child different ways to cope with intense feelings and to control their emotional reactions. This could involve teaching them relaxation strategies or problem-solving measures.

Promote Empathy: Encourage your child to understand the emotions of others. Show them how to empathize with other people's feelings.

In conclusion, promoting resilience and emotional intelligence in your child requires understanding, time, patience, and consistent efforts. Remember that every child is unique and what works for one may not work for another. Practice these strategies and modify them as needed to suit your child's unique needs and temperament.

Chapter 10. The Role of Empathy in No-Shame Parenting

Rising as the morning sun, the empathy in no-shame parenting showers a warm, soft light on the darker, colder aspects of traditional disciplinary measures. When a parent's response is governed by empathy, rather than by frustration, irritation, or anger, an environment of understanding, acceptance, and love is fostered.

10.1. Engaging with Empathy: The Basics

Empathy is the ability to understand and share the feelings of another. In the context of parenting, this means being cognizant of your child's emotions, thoughts, and experiences. Most parents love their children and believe they intuitively understand them. However, true empathy goes deeper than a simple gut feeling or instinct—it requires conscious effort, practice, awareness, and open-heartedness.

Empathy allows you to feel your child's struggle, not as an external observer but as if you're living it. This doesn't mean you should be engulfed by your child's emotions, but rather develop a profound understanding of their experience, which can offer the right support they need.

10.2. Setting the Stage for Empathy: Mindful Awareness

One of the first steps to becoming an empathetic parent is to cultivate mindful awareness of your own emotions. Often, parents react reflexively to their child's challenging behaviours out of frustration or exhaustion. These reactive responses usually stem from unobserved emotions and thought patterns.

To respond empathetically, start by taking a moment to pause and fully recognize your feelings. Are you feeling defensive? Overwhelmed? Irritated? Acknowledge these sensations without judgment. This is a challenging step, but it's essential in creating the emotional space required to respond effectively and empathetically to your child.

10.3. Walking in Their Tiny Shoes: Understanding Your Child's World

Children have their own perspectives, flashpoints, fears, and delights. Recognize that even as their parent, there will be gaps in your understanding of their world. Regularly communicate and listen to your child to gain new insights. Get down to their level—both physically and metaphorically—and validate their feelings. Use phrases like "It sounds like you're...", "I can see that you're feeling...", or "You seem...". These are incredibly powerful in expressing empathy.

Reluctance to acknowledge your child's difficult emotions might come from your own discomfort in facing similar emotions previously. Rather than try to fix the issue immediately, offer comfort and understanding.

10.4. A Powerful Tool: Empathetic Language

Language molds reality. Using empathetic language ensures your child feels heard and seen, that their feelings are legitimate and that they are not alone. Communicate with love and respect, voicing your own feelings and needs without blaming or criticizing. Steer clear of dismissive language like "Don't cry" or "You're overreacting".

Statements like "I understand you're upset because you wanted to keep playing, but it's bedtime now." validate feelings while reiterating the need for boundaries and rules.

10.5. Transforming Mistakes into Lessons: Embrace Imperfections

In a shame-free parenting approach, mistakes are seen not as character flaws but as opportunities to learn and grow. Empathy plays an enormous role here, as it allows parents to accept and understand their child's imperfections without blame or judgment. It's an opportunity to teach your child problem-solving skills and resilience in the face of failure, a valuable lesson that applies to both the child and parent.

Embracing imperfections and encouraging continuous growth helps build a safe space where children can express their feelings without the fear of negative criticism, fostering confidence, and individuality.

10.6. Empathy and Connection: Strengthening the Parent-Child Bond

Empathy, when practiced consistently, builds and strengthens the bond between parent and child. It encourages your child to come to you during their most vulnerable moments, knowing they will be met with understanding and love. It allows mutual trust to grow, offering your child the safety to express their emotions openly.

Overall, the role of empathy in no-shame parenting is a pervasive one. It is felt in every warm and understanding response, every loving and accepting conversation, every forgiving and patient moment. Through empathy, we can understand before we chastise, comfort before we criticize, and connect before we control. While traditional disciplinary measures attempt to mold children into preconceived boxes, empathy allows us to celebrate our children for who they truly are, fostering a household environment that is rich in understanding, acceptance, and love.

Chapter 11. Maintaining Balance: The Importance of Self-Care in Parenting

In the whirlwind of parenting, self-care is often pushed to the bottom of the pile. However, self-care needs to be more than just an afterthought: it's a necessity for maintaining a healthy balance and becoming the parent you aspire to be.

11.1. The Parenting Paradox

Parenting is a labor of love, thought, emotion, and energy. To figure out the balance between caring for your child and caring for yourself, you must first acknowledge the paradox. Everyone dispenses parental advice with the best of intentions, but it's vital to remember that what works for one may not for another. Many parental duties may leave you feeling drained, leaving little energy for self-care. However, neglecting your well-being can lead to burnout, impacting your ability to parent effectively.

11.2. Why Self-Care is Crucial

Let's begin by debunking the misconception that self-care is selfish. It's not. Caring for one's mental, physical, and emotional health, in fact, brings a positive influence on kids. When you are energized and emotionally resilient, it reflects on your everyday interaction with your children, thus paving the way for their healthier upbringing.

Moreover, you serve as a role model for your child. Adopting and demonstrating good self-care practices attributes to their understanding of the importance of personal health and well-being.

11.3. Unpacking Self-Care

If self-care seems nebulous, here is a three-pronged approach to break it down: physical self-care, emotional self-care, and spiritual self-care.

Physical self-care entails regular exercise, balanced diet, sufficient sleep, regular medical checkups, and perhaps, pampering yourself with a spa day once in a while. It also suggests saying no when you are overburdened or need rest.

Emotional self-care means acknowledging your feelings and giving yourself permission to experience them. It involves cultivating positive self-talk, seeking professional help if needed, and forming supportive social connections.

Spiritual self-care doesn't necessarily imply religion: it could also mean spending time in nature, practicing mindfulness, meditating, or engaging in activities that replenish your spirit.

11.4. Finding Your Version of Self-Care

As every individual is unique, self-care must be personalized. While some might find renewal in solitude, others might recharge by socializing. Some may resort to physical activities, others to art or music. Thus, define your self-care and find what rejuvenates you–be it a walk in the park, a yoga session, or just an uninterrupted cup of coffee.

Understand that you might not always have large chunks of time at your disposal. Incorporating small practices throughout the day, like deep breathing or momentary pauses, can also contribute significantly to your well-being.

Initiatives such as journaling or maintaining a gratitude log might also help elevate emotional health.

11.5. Setting Boundaries

Setting healthy boundaries — both with your children and others around you — is essential for maintaining balance. Make your children understand that parents need their personal space and time. Simultaneously, teach them about the importance of boundaries and personal space for themselves, fostering a baseline for their future relationships.

11.6. Cultivating a Support Network

Reach out to friends, family, or local community groups to create a strong support network. This network can facilitate shared parenting responsibilities and provide you the much-needed breather.

Online platforms, too, offer an array of parenting forums where you can connect with parents across the globe, share experiences, and gain insights.

11.7. Seek Professional Help If Needed

If you ever feel persistently low or overwhelmed, do not hesitate to seek professional help. Mental health is as crucial as physical health, and sometimes, therapy or counseling might provide the necessary tools for navigating through difficult phases.

11.8. Final Takeaway

Self-care in parenting is not a luxury; it's a necessity. It's about creating a sustainable system that maintains your health and happiness while fulfilling your responsibilities as a parent. The journey of self-care is ongoing: you might experience hiccups along the way, but remember, it's about progress, not perfection.

Embrace self-care, and witness the transformation it brings not only to you, but also to the way you parent and the environment you create for your child. Ensuring your well-being is, indirectly, one of the best gifts you can give your child.